Your
Aging Parents

◆

For my mother

◆

Your Aging Parents

Allison Greene

Smyth & Helwys Publishing, Inc.
Macon, GA

ISBN 1-57312-013-8

Your Aging Parents
Allison Greene

©1995
Smyth & Helwys Publishing, Inc.®
6316 Peake Road
Macon, Georgia 31210-3960
1-800-568-1248

Library of Congress Cataloging-in-Publication Data

Greene, Allison.
    Your aging parents / by Allison Greene.
       ix + 78pp.   5.5" x 8.5 (14 x 21.5 cm.)
    Includes bibliographical references.
    ISBN 1-57312-013-8
    1. Aging parents. 2. Parent and adult child. 3. Aged—
Family relationships. I. Title.
HQ1063.6.G744   1995
306.874—dc20
                               95–16192
                                     CIP

Contents

Preface

Getting started on this book was a difficult endeavor for me. I did not anticipate how hard it would be. A few months ago, I led a six-week course at our church on "Understanding Aging Parents." Various church members came up to me and said, "I wish we could have gotten to the sessions. They would have been very helpful to our group." These comments prompted me to consider the possibility of putting the information into a book for their use after the workshop.

When I proposed the idea to the editors at Smyth and Helwys, they said yes to the idea. Since then, every time I have mentioned the book-in-progress to the groups I lead, their response has been: "I can't wait to read that!" "Hurry up!" "I need it!" "What about commitment (incompetency) issues?" "Tell us what to do!"

That is when I balk. Even though I have dealt with the issue of caring for aging parents both personally and professionally for many years, I cannot tell you what to do. What an intimidating, terrifying thought! I certainly do not have the answers to what is likely to be the gravest issue we as a society have to face. With all of its multiple implications—and each individual with his/her many layers of emotions—there is no one answer to apply to a person's unique situation.

What we do have is each other. There are common threads in this experience. In this book you will find my story along with practical information: what to be aware of, how to access help, how to know and choose your options. There is also permission to feel and claim your emotions and encouragement to share them.

The activities at the end of each chapter are geared to group discussion or personal exploration. They are intended to increase your understanding of the complexity of the

aging issue, to offer further avenues of help and information, and to challenge you to find your own redemptive
healing along with others in the process. You will find it
helpful to share your story; soon you will realize that the
stories of others in your group are not so different from
your own. Godspeed!

Allison Greene

Acknowledgments

Special thanks to

my family: Vic, Megan, and John

encouraging friends, especially Baxter Wynn, Margaret Brissey, and Roger Gower, for keeping me going on this endeavor

those who participated in the leadership of the initial six-week sessions

other professionals who reviewed the content: Cassandra E. Bray, M.D.; Lesley R. Moore, Esquire; Valerie Peterson, R.N., M.N., C.S.; and Paul H. Grier

co-workers who endured my stress

a place at 300 Pettigru to put it all together

Chapter 1

Beginning the Process

My job of caring for an aging parent began with a phone call. It was about 7:30 P.M., and we were just finishing dinner.

"I've been having these pains all in my chest and down my arm for the past several hours. Maybe it was from the lunch today. I cannot eat those fancy foods; but it seems to be getting worse. I thought I should let someone know," said my mother.

Two days earlier, we had taken Mother out for her birthday. She looked lovely, her slender frame clothed in a soft green suit. She held the hand of each grandchild with hers as we entered the restaurant. Healthy throughout my thirty-four years, she kept my pre-schooler weekday afternoons and frequently cooked supper for us. While she had been widowed for five years, she still drove to nearby activities, managed her house and finances, taught Sunday school in a nursing home, and often told me what to do.

The evening of her call, my husband went over to her house, which was only three blocks away, to check on her. As is typical of those in the "sandwich generation," who must care for the old and the young, we had two children who could not be left alone. I was also having some health problems and, to add to the stress, I had recently quit my job to go into business for myself. This particular decision became a significant factor later on in the process with regard to financial strain and taking off time from work.

The hospital decided to keep Mother overnight for observation. Then another call came at about 5:00 A.M. This time the call was from the hospital asking me to come quickly.

"No!" I remember saying out loud after hanging up. "I'm not ready!"

Two nurses were waiting for me when I reached the critical care unit. "We need some medical history on her," they said. "When was she last hospitalized?"

"When I was born . . . ," I replied, ". . . in 1953."

They found it hard to believe she was eighty-two, and kept commenting on how sweet she was.

Sweet? I nearly laughed. The rigid, opinionated, worrying, controlling, powerful person I had grown up with? Strong, maybe; smart, determined, and demanding, definitely; loving, yes, but sweet?

Then I remembered Saturday mornings when I was little. Saturday was the only day the family did not have to rush anywhere. Mother would get into the wide sunlit bed with me, laugh, and read me Robert Louis Stevenson, Little Women, *and Bible stories. When I later read* Gone with the Wind *and Shakespeare, they were her hardback copies from the 1930s.*

I remember being scared of the dark and crying out, "Tell me a story, Mama. Not a made-up one; one about when you were little." And she would begin, "One afternoon I went out into the pasture where I was not supposed to go, because Papa kept the bulls there. And this bull calf got after me and butted me down the hill! I crawled through the fence, but my arm hurt so bad! I thought it was broken. I didn't want to tell

Mama 'cause she would scold me. So I hid and cried behind the shed."

"What happened, Mama?" I asked, rubbing my own arm.

"Long about suppertime, Mama came looking for me and heard me crying. She took me up to the house and looked after my arm."

"She didn't fuss?"

"Not that time. Your Granny loved us—all her own ten children and four of our cousins who stayed every summer— but she could not show it very well. Now get to sleep!"

And I would give into sleep, living those stories and breathing the strength of who my mother was.

"The doctor is in with her now," the nurse told me. "She was doing fine, then something happened. Her blood pressure bottomed out, and we started losing her. We have changed the medication and are waiting to see if that helps."

Oh, God.

"You can come on in, " she added.

I stood in the corner of the small white and chrome cubicle while two nurses and a doctor moved around her. Trained as a medical social worker, I was used to being backstage in crisis situations—just not with my mother.

"She's beginning to stabilize," the doctor said. "We will be close by."

I was then alone with her for a few moments. As I approached the bed, I noticed that her figure looked shriveled in the shapeless hospital gown; her hair was disarrayed. She moved restlessly, groaning and speaking incoherently.

"Mother," I took her hand, "I'm here."

"What is on your face?" she asked, grasping the air and trying to catch something. "Don't you see them?"

"It's the medicine, Mama. It's O.K." I gave her some cracked ice.

"Bathroom," she said. "I want to go to the bathroom." I looked around for the metal pan and tried to place it correctly for her.

I don't like this, but why is helping your mother go to the bathroom so different from helping your child? As I emptied the bed pan, the walls of the room seemed to close in on me, and I felt dizzy. I wished that one of the nurses would return. If it is the hospital's policy that there be no visitors permitted in CCU, then why do they want me back here? I am afraid to know the answer.

Mother, however, rallied. They moved her to a room after a few days and prepared her for heart catherization. She was ready. "You know, lots of people have that by-pass surgery," she said, "and they do just fine." I did not feel as optimistic. For once, I was right.

In Mother's case, significantly blocked arteries—too brittle for surgery—caused her heart attack, consequent failing health, and eventual dementia. For the next three-and-a-half years, we passed through various stages of caregiving. Each stage was different, distinct, and emotionally and physically difficult for everyone involved.

In many ways I felt like I had been preparing to care for aging parents most of my life. My parents were in their late forties when I was born; I was their only child. When I was four, my father had a major heart attack, leaving him a semi-invalid until his death twenty-five years later. He could never pick me up after the first heart attack. The experience with my father was the beginning of role reversal for me, as well as a fear that the world was a scary place. From my earliest memories, I recall having a sense of need to take care of my parents.

This eventually led me to studying gerontology in graduate school and working with older persons as a hospital social worker. It was not until my mother's heart attack and my being actively involved with her daily care until her death, that I really lived it.

I learned many lessons. What I remember most was feeling dead tired and inadequate to everyone in my life. I also found that there was no one to talk to, no one who could understand, and no time to try to explain it. Mine was an isolating experience. My friends, like my husband, had healthy parents still active in their sixties. They had siblings and the privilege of still being "children." Their focus was on developing their careers, or being involved in their children's lives, or both. They were not having to get their parents to the bathroom, or clean out the house of their childhood, or make excruciating decisions for other people's lives. My friends could be involved in church and volunteer work; they could laugh, and play, and even take vacations.

Now with hindsight, I can see consolation. Although I may have been younger than most persons on the curve of dealing with aging parents, I was not alone. The various stages I experienced were not unique to me. In fact, they are becoming increasingly more common to many of us. How well we deal with these stages is determined to a large extent by how much information we have available to us, how prepared we are, and how well we share and process our feelings with those who can understand.

Aging as Process

Being old is a state of being and of oldness. We often
forget that being is becoming, and the emphasis on old
may overshadow being. 'Being' holds endless potential
at any moment, whereas 'old' implies finite and the end.
If one's eyes are on the end rather than each moment of
being, despair ensues. A future orientation is attributed
to the young and a past orientation to the old, but a present orientation is needed for full living at any age.[1]

Although most of us do not look forward to growing
older, our choices are rather limited. Aging happens to all
of us—to us and to our parents. The process of aging is not
something we can halt, fix, or control. What many of us in
our American youth-and-beauty conscious culture seem to
forget is that aging is a process, a naturally occurring part
of living. For most of us, however, aging often sneaks up
on us. I overheard a conversation the other day between
two men. "What really bothers me about turning seventy,"
said one man, "is that Daddy died at seventy." "I know
what you mean," replied the other. "I remember Dad had
his heart attack when he was fifty-eight, and I thought he
was *ancient*."

A survey conducted by *PARADE Magazine* found that
older Americans have fewer fears and less negative views
of aging than do younger people.[2] Also, the older the
respondents, the older the age they defined as "old." Older
persons did not see themselves as old, regardless of whether they were 65, 75, or 85. Among those age 65 to 75, only
14 percent responded that they had a negative view of
aging. In fact, the fear of aging seems to decrease with

aging, with 85 percent of that group saying they were not afraid of getting old.

Few people, however, would say that getting old is easy. Often older persons face declining health, limited resources, and various losses. Losses experienced as one gets older include the loss of a long-time companion, physical abilities or even mental faculties, separation from children and other loved ones, and the loss of independence. How individuals respond to these unwanted changes seems to be unique but never easy.

The old are getting older, and there are increasingly more of them. According to the U.S. Census Bureau, the number of Americans 65 or older will increase from 31 million in 1990 to 40 million by 2010. The oldest segment of this group, those 85-plus, will grow even more quickly: from 3.1 million to 5.7 million. How will these individuals —our grandparents, our parents, *ourselves*—be cared for? That is the crucial question facing our society today.

Rosalynn Carter in her book, *Helping Yourself Help Others*, recalls Margaret Mead's remark that a society is judged on the way it treats its elderly.[3] Traditionally in some societies, older members have been revered. In others, the aged have simply walked off into the wilderness, to face death privately and alone. Although this route may still appeal to some persons today, it is not very practical or possible.

While in America the focus has been more on the younger generation, this trend may be changing with the "graying" of America. The largest segment of the population—the Baby Boomers, those born between the years of 1946 and 1963—faces caring for aging parents and, soon, themselves. Our current older population has become a powerful force in government and legislative issues.

Membership in the American Association of Retired Persons was 34,000,000 in 1994.

Even now, at age 40, I start to worry about getting old. My hips ache after a light run, my knees hurt when I climb the stairs, gray hairs appear more frequently, and my skin is not as wrinkle-free. How we deal with the aging process begins with each of us, early in life. As a society we need to turn to our elders in their wisdom of life to learn how to grow old.

Activities

Activity I: There are many misunderstandings about aging and older people. Take the following quiz to find out how much you know.[4] Then discuss with some of those in your group the findings that surprised you. (Answers to quiz in Appendix A.)

Aging: Myth versus Fact

1. The majority of older people (over age 65) are senile.
2. All five senses tend to decline in old age.
3. Most old people have no interest in or capacity for sexual relations.
4. Lung capacity tends to decline in old age.
5. The majority of old people feel miserable most of the time.
6. Physical strength tends to decline in old age.
7. At least one-tenth of the aged are living in long-term care institutions.

8. Aged drivers have fewer accidents per person than drivers under age 65.
9. Most older workers cannot work as effectively as younger workers.
10. About 80 percent of the aged are healthy enough to carry out their normal activities.
11. Most older people are set in their ways and unable to change.
12. Old people usually take longer to learn something.
13. It is almost impossible for most older people to learn something new.
14. The reaction of most older people tends to be slower than the reaction of younger people.
15. In general, most older people are pretty much alike.
16. The majority of older people are seldom bored.
17. The majority of older people are socially isolated and lonely.
18. Older workers have fewer accidents than younger workers.
19. Over 15 percent of the U.S. population is now age 65 or over.
20. Most medical practitioners tend to give low priority to the aged.
21. The majority of older people have incomes below the poverty level (as defined by the federal government).
22. The majority of older people are working or would like to have some kind of work to do (including housework or volunteer work).
23. Older people tend to become more religious as they age.
24. Most older people are seldom irritated or angry.

25. The health and socioeconomic status of older people (compared to younger people) in the year 2000 will probably be about the same as now.

Activity II: Many older persons experience stress in their daily living. Consider the following suggestions and share them with your parents to help them stay healthy and independent.[5]

Stay Involved and Active

- Get involved in community affairs.
- Volunteer.
- Take classes at local colleges or community centers.
- Join a group of peers in a social group or a support group.
- Make it a rule to visit with family and friends.
- Encourage and accept help from others.
- Stay in touch with others through telephone calls, letters, and visits.
- Invite others to your home.
- Listen to the radio or TV call-in programs and participate in community affairs.
- Find out about community resources.

Deal with Your Feelings

- Accept that there are many times when you may feel sad or angry.
- Discuss your feelings with others.

- Treat yourself; each day focus on simple pleasures (a favorite food, T. V. show, or hobby).
- Be easy on yourself; don't expect perfection.
- Give yourself credit for the things you accomplish, no matter how small.
- Balance your responsibilities and interests.
- Make whatever form of relaxation that works for you a regular part of your life.

Learn to Relax

- Keep faithful to a practical exercise program.
- Learn to meditate.
- Do things you enjoy.
- Enjoy your home.
- Listen to music.

Maintain Good Health Habits

- Have regular physical exams.
- Exercise regularly.
- Eat a balanced diet.
- Get enough sleep.
- Avoid alcohol.
- Be careful about taking drugs, both prescription and over-the-counter.
- Get help when you need it.

Activity III: A living will, or advanced directives, is a document that most older persons will want to have ready. In fact, a living will is important for persons of any age.

Hospitals are now required by law to have one for each patient. If a person is not capable of completing the form upon admission, the next of kin must make decisions for the patient. In an emergency situation where no living will is available, full life-support measures will be initiated. In this case, these measures may need to be discontinued at a later date.

Complete a living will for yourself, and then ask your parents about theirs. This step is an important one to take in preparing for the future.

Further Exploration
◆Individually or in a group◆

Exploration I: Write your own thoughts as to how you see yourself at age 65 or 75 or 85. What will you be doing? How will you feel? What would you desire your situation to be like?

Exploration II: Read the children's book, *Love You Forever.*[6] What feelings does the book evoke?

Exploration III: Visit an older person and try to view the process of living from his or her perspective.

Exploration IV: Challenge yourself to remain aware of legislation affecting older persons. Remember, it will matter to you, too!

Notes

[1]B. Steffl, *Handbook of Gerontological Nursing* (New York, NY: VanNostrand-Reinhold,1884) 103.

[2]Mark Clements, "What We Say About Aging," *PARADE Magazine* (12 Dec 1993) 4.

[3]Rosalynn Carter, *Helping Yourself Help Others* (New York: Random House, 1994) 14.

[4]Adapted from Erdman Palmore, "Facts on Aging: A Short Quiz," *The Gerontologist* (August 1977) 315–316.

[5]Reprinted from AARP's Caregivers in the Workplace Kit.

[6]Robert Munsch, *Love You Forever* (Ontario: Firefly Books Ltd., 1986).

Chapter 2

Coping with Sources of Stress

"You have five major blockages, Sara," the doctor told my mother after the heart catherization. "One artery is totally occluded, one 95 percent, and the other 90 percent. I have consulted with our heart specialist, and surgery is not an option."

"But I'm willing to try it," she insisted.

"It's not that," he responded. "At your age, the vessels are just too brittle. I'm sorry." He left, and she was quiet, quieter than I ever remembered.

The doctor waited for me in the hall. "It does not look good, but with care she will be all right for awhile."

"How long?" I asked.

"A year, maybe three at the most. I do not want her walking much; no hills or stairs and no driving. She should stay on her diet, and do nothing that upsets her. Now, she's going home with you, right?"

"For now, anyway," I said, knowing that I would do whatever I could to take care of her.

So Mother came to our three-bedroom, two-child, and two-career home. The first three weeks she was quiet, and we all waited on her. The children tiptoed cautiously around her. I checked on her during the night, helped her to the bathroom, monitored her medications, and cooked her special diet. In addition to Mother's care, I was trying to survive in a new business, finish graduate school, help with homework, and get to soccer games.

During the next several weeks Mother's condition improved. She alienated the sitter and complained that I did not get home soon enough, worked too hard, neglected the children, and did not eat enough.

On the sixth Sunday I broke down when my daughter —echoing her grandmother's words and tone—chastened me for not spending enough time with her. I went to my bed in tears and could not get up. Then, my mother made the decision to go. She moved back to her house with a live-in helper at night, received Meals-on-Wheels at noon, and was checked on regularly by our family.

The following year, Mother's condition reflected less noticeable changes. I scheduled the surgery I had postponed earlier, even though part of me was afraid she would die before I could recover.

Mother's condition remained stable. She was even able to come over and stay with me when I returned home from the hospital. She made chicken salad, hot rolls, and jello. Once again—at least for a while—she took care of me. I began my process of preparation.

Common Sources of Stress

In many ways, the initial six-week experience of Mother living with us was like a microcosm for the rest of our time. The weeks caring for her were full of many identifiable stressors. Although I was not conscious of them at the time—much less able to deal with them—an awareness had begun. Throughout the following months I was able to see many elements that made the task of caring for an aging parent even more difficult. Such difficulties included my life-long relationship with my mother, relationships with immediate and extended family, physical circumstances, and financial situations.

The parent-child relationship is the oldest and strongest bond a person can experience; more often than not, it is full of conflict and pain. As parents, we want *everything* for our children; as children, we would do anything to please our parents. The expectations on both sides, however, are frequently met with frustration, hurt, disappointment, and anger. Recognizing the many emotions brought to such a significant relationship may help in dealing with the stresses that are intensified by external factors.

In my case, my mother had always had high expectations for me. I was born to her during her mid-years and was her only child—the only egg in her basket! I remember, with bitterness, her sighing with disappointment when I brought home papers from school with a grade of "98" or "99." "Oh," she would say, "it was almost a '100.' "

Maybe Mother did not mean this nearly as seriously as I internalized it. These perceptions, however, contributed to my adult expectations of perfection and my driving need to achieve and succeed in everything I attempted. Not long after my Mother's death, I realized that she really only wanted me to be happy. Her aging drove me even harder to prove myself, or to be good enough—before it was too late. During the years when she was in need of care, I was in a desperate struggle myself: to finish graduate school, run a business, and have the perfect home and family. It

was a dual battle we were unable to share. I heard her crit-
icisms; she saw my busyness.

My mother and I were never able to communicate well.
As early as adolescence, I had learned to deal with her
constant critique by keeping my feelings hidden and a
smile on my face. She was always able to converse, but not
about things such as love or death. She often told me what
to do; I pretended never to hear. If we could have learned
the skill of listening to one another, the last stages might
not have been as difficult and lonely for either of us.

Family Relationships

When change affects one member of a family, it affects all
members. Since I was an only child, I felt the sole responsibility of my mother's care. In talking with many children
who care for aging parents, however, it seems that the
caregiving responsibility falls primarily on one member
anyway. This responsibility usually falls on a daughter,
which is why many researchers say that the caregiving role
is primarily a women's issue. One child may live closer,
while others are far away. Often there is disagreement
between siblings as to what is needed and how it will be
done. Anger, guilt, and lack of communication are common
among siblings and within the parent/child relationship.

In the caregiver's nuclear family, relations are also
strained. While my husband was helpful and supportive, I
never felt he could really understand. Sometimes it made
me mad that he dared to try! When he had to accept a
greater role in caring for our children—the elementary
school crowd called him "mother of the year"—I felt

resentment because I could not be as involved as I would have liked to during this time.

Although our children were young and they loved their grandmother very much, they too felt the stress. Their schedules and patterns were disrupted and their routines were interrupted. Three-generational families are not what we have become accustomed to as a society. We are more familiar with soccer games and fast food, longer working hours and an accelerated pace, and children who have become louder and more outspoken.

More women work outside the home than ever before. In the more typical "sandwich generation" scenario, there are teenagers at home, an additional strain of caring for adolescence and aging parents. Older children—those sixty-five years and above—facing their own health problems and limited incomes, may be caring for parents in their eighties and beyond.

Extended family members can become involved as well, often by placing additional demands on the primary care-giver to *do something!* Often they do not understand that nothing else can be done for the parent. Extended family members may be concerned because their relative is chang-ing and may want you to "fix" things over which you have no control. Sometimes members of the family will want you to ignore situations about your parent because they do not want to face the reality themselves.

Fortunately, I had an extended family who listened when I called, who helped in the intervention with my mother, and who supported me throughout the process. Not everyone is so lucky.

Physical Settings
and Financial Situations

Physical and financial circumstances are also significant. Not every home is equipped to care for an aging person, and many homes do not have a downstairs sleep space or bath. While few families can afford to move or make costly renovations, most older people (83 percent) say they would never want to live with their children.

Financial matters always seem to be a major stress factor. Adult children may be struggling with careers, families, and mortgages. Some caregivers may be paying for children in college or even trying to set aside something for their own retirement. Aging parents are living on a fixed income and fear that their savings will not be enough. Recent projections show that these savings will more than likely not be enough. "Even those who have sizable nest eggs will become destitute after two years in a long-term care facility," some experts direly predict.[1] And, "that same length of time impoverishes over half of the families providing care at home to Alzheimer's patients."[2]

Insurance companies are reluctant to offer substantial elder care policies because sound actuarial estimates of long-term care are not readily calculable. More and more, children may be contributing to their parents' care. There are already tax allowances in place and provisions in scholarship programs that shelter income for caring for aging parents. Long-term care may be a greater expense than any of us can bear.

Financial advisors can offer suggestions and creative solutions for what may work best for the financial situation of yourself and your parents. Often parents will begin divesting possessions to their children. Attorneys can assist in providing guidelines and establishing protections for the older person.

Activities

Activity I: Stay aware of your personal stress level. Complete the following "Stress Test" (Social Readjustment Rating Scale).[3] Discuss your scores and high stress areas. Note that for a score over 300, there is more than an 80 percent chance of a stress-related illness. Learn to take care of yourself!

Event	Value	Score
1. Death of spouse	100	
2. Divorce	73	
3. Marital separation	65	
4. Jail term	63	
5. Death of a close family member	63	
6. Personal injury of illness	53	
7. Marriage	50	
8. Fired from work	47	
9. Marital reconciliation	45	
10. Retirement	44	
11. Change in family member's health	40	
12. Pregnancy	39	
13. Sex difficulties	39	
14. Addition to family	39	
15. Business readjustment	39	

16. Change in financial status   38
17. Death of a close friend   37
18. Change to different line of work   36
19. Change in number of marital
    arguments   36
20. Debt over $10,000   35
21. Foreclosure of mortgage or loan   31
22. Change in work responsibilities   30
23. Son or daughter leaving home   29
24. Trouble with in-laws   29
25. Outstanding personal
    achievement   29
26. Spouse begins or stops work   28
27. Starting or finishing school   26
28. Change in living conditions   26
29. Revision of personal habits   25
30. Trouble with boss   24
31. Change in work hours, conditions   23
32. Change in residence   20
33. Change in schools   20
34. Change in recreational habits   20
35. Change in religious activities   19
36. Change in social activities   19
37. Loan under $10,000   18
38. Change in sleeping habits   17
39. Change in number of family
    gatherings   16
40. Change in eating habits   15
41. Vacation   13
42. Christmas/holiday season   12
43. Minor violation of law   11

Activity II: How well do you acknowledge and communicate your feelings? Generate discussion about those feelings that are hard for you to express. Share ideas about how to accept all of our feelings. Consider forming a support group in your church or community to focus on the issue of caring for aging parents.

Activity III: Since most older people say they never want to be dependent on their children, some gerontologists believe our society will see an increase in assisted suicides and suicide pacts among older persons. What do you think? How can we affect the issue of euthanasia?

Further Exploration
◆Individually or in a group◆

Exploration I: Along with your parent(s), consult a lawyer and/or financial advisor about planning for the future. Make sure wills are in order. Establish joint signatures on bank accounts and initiate a durable power of attorney. Talk to your parents about important decisions that may have to be made in their future. Give them the opportunity to tell you their wishes.

Exploration II: Begin now (or continue) the process of understanding yourself and your relationship to parents. Ask your minister or counselor for assistance, read books, and visit support groups.

Notes

[1]David Haber, *Health Care for an Aging Society* (New York: Hemisphere Publishing, Co., 1989) 22.
[2]Ibid.
[3]T. H. Holmes and R. H. Rahe, "The Social Readjustment Rating Scale," *Journal of Psychosomatic Research* (11 April 1967): 213–218.

Chapter 3

Noticing the Changes

A siren pierced the late afternoon traffic sounds. "It's a fire truck!" "No, it's an ambulance." My two children argued back and forth.

"There it is," said my sitter as we entered my mother's street. A woman lay on the side of the road. I saw her brown walking shoes first and then her striped sweater.

"It's Mother," I said, thinking she was dead. I drove past the ambulance and jerked to a stop a half-block away in front of her house. Ordering the children to stay in the car, I ran toward the small clustered group, screaming, "It's my mother!"

"It's O.K.!" called a neighbor. "They don't think it's her heart! She just fell!"

She was lying on her back. Her eyes were open, blood was pouring from her forehead; at least she was conscious. Attendants were getting the stretcher ready. She looked up at me and, only slightly bemused, she asked, "What are you doing here?"

"I was just driving by taking Edna home," I responded.

"I do not know what happened," she said. "I was walking right along, and all of a sudden I was going down, down, down."

"I'll meet you at the hospital," I called as they loaded her into the ambulance. Running back to the children, I explained, "I have to go to the hospital with Marmee. Let's go in the house and call Ellen to come get you. Tell Daddy to come to the hospital."

Briefly aware of reaching for the familiar key and fitting it into the heavy white door, I hurried in. Nothing was different: celery green carpet in the hall, blue speckled linoleum and dark red counter tops in the kitchen, and everything in its place. Thirty-two years had passed since my father built the house. The house had experienced many departures: I left at age 20, then my father's death at age 78, and now my mother at age 83. Many times during the past year I had entered the house with trepidation, fearful of her failing condition.

The emergency room was crowded at 5:30 P.M., but nurses carried her straight back. Her vital signs were fine; she had a broken shoulder. We were left alone in the curtained-drawn cubicle—she on the cold chrome table, I on the round metal stool. There we waited; for over six hours we waited. They gave her nothing for the pain. Finally, someone brought a blanket to help stop her shivering.

"Where is the doctor?" I demanded.

"He has several patients that are more critical ahead of her. He'll be here soon," replied a nurse.

Mother lay very calmly, only moaning when anything moved her left arm. "Does it hurt?" I asked.

"Not too bad," Mother responded.

So we waited, she in and out of mild shock and I watching and listening to the "more critical" around us. There was a man who had split his head open in a motorcycle accident, a boy with a smashed pelvis, and a young

woman with a broken hip. I also noticed—in the cold gray corridor beside X-ray—an old man with sunken cheeks and thin arms who had been brought in alone from a nursing home. He mumbled and waved for me.
I made out his words. "So nice," he said, nodding toward my mother. "She has someone with her."
In X-ray the technicians could not get the angle right. They tried again and again until Mother blacked out. I ran for a resident.
"Calm down," he told me. "She'll be fine." Then he walked off.
I wished him old and helpless and alone.
By midnight it was over, and I was told to take her home.

Physical Changes

A fact of aging is that our bodies experience wear over time. Many of our senses begin to dull, joints hurt, and processes slow down. Although the aging process usually begins at about age 40, the greatest amount of total health care dollars is spent during the last two years of an older person's life. Being aware of and noticing changes in an aging parent's health can make it easier to understand what is happening in the process.

◆*Vision loss* is customary with aging. Besides needing bifocal lenses or reading glasses, older persons may have difficulty seeing at night and judging distances. These changes can impact their ability to drive, read medication instructions, see whether a stove burner is on or off, recognize people, or even move around safely. The inability to see clearly can also affect the cleanliness of surroundings and personal hygiene.

Three common disorders of the eyes are *retinal disease, glaucoma, and cataracts.* Regular check-ups by eye-care professionals are extremely important for older people. When detected early, the effects of these disorders can be minimized or corrected with minor surgery.

As the eyes age, older persons may experience *dry eyes* and *blurred vision.* Colors may be less distinct and harder to differentiate. More intense light may be needed to see, glare is more pronounced, depth perception is decreased, and adaptation to dark and light is hindered. The older person may also be less aware of injury or infection because of *decreased corneal sensitivity.*

Bright lights, vivid colors, large print books, and even books on tape can help the older person compensate for some of these vision changes.

♦*Hearing loss* in aging can result from many causes, and hearing aids are not always the simple remedy. *Neural loss* may not be helped by amplifying the sound; instead, increased ringing and clashing of sound can occur. Older persons need to be evaluated by a hearing specialist to determine what is possible to augment their hearing ability. *Assistive devices* or *flashing lights* may need to be installed on telephones.

Some conditions of the ear that result from aging are:

- increased production and thickness of ear wax
- hair growth in the auditory canal
- loss of hair cells in the inner ear.

These conditions diminish hearing, particularly high-pitched sounds and voices.

Hearing loss impacts the older person's ability to communicate, understand instructions, and stay connected in a rapidly changing living environment. Older persons with hearing loss *can be mistaken as being confused, mis-diagnosed with dementia, or perceived to be willfully contrary.*

♦*Taste sensitivity* may also diminish with age. Often older people complain that nothing tastes good anymore. They tend to prefer sweets and more highly seasoned foods. Signs of a decrease in the sense of taste are:

- lower secretion of saliva
- a fissuring and furrowing of the tongue
- decreased oral sensation to hot and cold
- diminished thirst
- less efficient gag reflex.

Some implications for health and safety that are important to keep in mind are weight loss or malnutrition, increased sodium intake, poor oral hygiene, mouth irritation, dehydration, and choking or aspiration.

♦*Smell.* The sense of *smell* dulls with aging, most likely due to environmental factors such as smoking, occupational odors, and airborne pollutants. Changes in the mucous membranes result in nasal irritation, sneezing, and post nasal drip.

Diminished smell can cause weight loss or malnutrition, poor hygiene, and the inability to distinguish burning, spoiled foods, or gas fumes.

♦*Touch.* The sense of *touch* is not as sharp, thus making the simple task of picking up coins or fingering papers difficult. This sense also relates to the older person's *integument*, or outer covering of skin. Because the skin *grows less elastic* with age, it tears more easily. There is also less tolerance to the cold. The skin becomes drier, perspires less, and is more susceptible to bruising and burns. Hair on all parts of the body thins considerably.

Health risks relating to the sense of touch are as follows:

- hypothermia
- skin tears and pressure sores
- dehydration and heat exhaustion
- accidental burning and other hazards
- and poorer absorption of subcutaneous drugs.

Older persons may feel *temperature discomforts* during bathing, dressing, or medical exams. Systems within the body show signs of the aging process as well. Some of the effects are:

- **Neurologic**—Slower reaction time; decreased short-term memory; decline in problem-solving ability; poorer quality of sleep; reduced recovery from stressors: heat, cold, and exercise; older persons may experience tremors associated with disease (such as Parkinson's).

- **Musculo-skeletal**—A sense of balance and coordination decreases; bones become more porous; difficulty in walking. Muscle atrophy causes increased abdominal girth and decreased weight. Ligaments lose elasticity causing stiff joints, wide gait with shuffling steps, and slower walking speed.

- **Gastro-intestinal**—Decrease in size of stomach and liver with poorer absorption of food and vitamins; constipation; reduced metabolism and needed caloric intake; decreased motility of esophagus, making swallowing difficult.

- **Genitourinary**—Bladder capacity decreases; stress incontinence; male prostate glands enlarge, causing increased risk of infection and obstruction; hormonal changes in women and increased infection risk in the urethra and bladder, often without fever or other typical symptoms.

- **Cardiovascular**—Increased arrhythmia; strength of heart muscle contraction decreases; less elasticity of vessels; increased systolic blood pressure.

- **Endocrine**—Decreased thyroid function can result in fatigue, depression, and confusion; glucose metabolism decreases because of lessened insulin release.

- **Respiratory**—Decreased protection of the central airway due to widening of the trachea; lungs larger because of decreasing elasticity; rib cage more rigid; airways tend to collapse when breathing is at low volumes and when lying down; increased risks of aspiration, choking, and pneumonia.

Mental Changes

The older person can experience mental changes, ranging from mild depression to severe dementia. Terms frequently used are explained on the following pages.

◆*Depression* can occur from many causes, such as the *multiple losses*—ability to drive or live independently—associated with aging. The older person may *lose pleasure* in activities and complain of headaches or fatigue.

◆*Delirium* is an acute, short-term condition, usually caused by infection or medication. In most cases the person's conditions improves over time. Delirium is common during acute illnesses or hospitalization.

◆*Dementia* is a group of symptoms that characterize certain conditions. Major symptoms involve a *decline in intellectual functioning* severe enough to interfere with routine activities. Alzheimer's disease is the most common form of dementia.

Alzheimer's begins slowly, usually with the older person not being able to find the right word or repeating the same question. The Alzheimer's patient may write many reminder notes, wear the same clothes day after day, and forget to pay bills or take medications. Later he or she may not be able to write or speak, recognize people, or chew and swallow. Becoming bedridden and incontinent, the Alzheimer's patient eventually loses consciousness, requires total care, and finally stops breathing. The disease affects some 7 to 9 percent of those persons age 65 and older, has *no known cure or cause*, and is *irreversible*. The disease may last anywhere from three to twenty years.

One researcher described the disease like this: "Dementia is like death. It is the death of the mind. Most family members will go through some phase of mourning that is often more grievous than that produced by the death itself."[1]

Caring for the Alzheimer's patient has been called "the thirty-six-hour day," which is also the title of a comprehensive and practical caregivers' handbook.[2] As the disease progresses, other caregivers must become involved in the process of caring for the aging parent. Whether the assistance comes from *respite care, adult daycare,* or *a nursing home,* the family will need to make decisions that are in the best interest of all involved. Alzheimer's is perhaps the primary illness where the parent-child roles become completely reversed.

Alzheimer's disease is the *third most costly disease* in the United States today. A study based on 1991 figures determined mid-range direct medical and social service costs at $47,581 per patient over the course of the disease. The total annual cost, including lost earnings and productivity, for 1994 was estimated at $82.7 billion.

◆*Senility* is a label often used to describe persons over age 65 having dementia. Now physicians recognize that senile dementia is not a normal process of aging but rather the result of a disease such as Alzheimer's.

◆*Chronic organic brain syndrome* is a term sometimes applied to persons with symptoms such as memory loss, disorientation, confusion, personality changes, and inability to carry out normal functions. Again, dementia is now considered the more accurate term.

◆*Hardening of the arteries, or arteriosclerosis,* is a symptom of dementia following the occurrence of strokes.

Anyone with symptoms of dementia should have a complete evaluation including:

- a physical, psychiatric, and neurological evaluation
- a detailed medical history
- a mental status test
- a neurological testing
- blood work and urinalysis
- a chest x-ray, EEG, CT scan, and EKG.

The evaluation will help determine whether the dementia is the result of a treatable illness. In most cases, the evaluation is about 90 percent accurate. (The only way to confirm a diagnosis of Alzheimer's disease is by autopsy.)

Activities
♦Individually or in a group♦

Activity I: Pair up with another member of your group and open the kit provided for you. One person will need to put on the pair of latex gloves, insert plugs in both ears, and wear the dark glasses. The other person will begin by handing the first person small objects such as a cotton ball, an alcohol toilette, and a bandaid. Ask your partner to tell you what the items are. Then talk with each other about what the experience felt like.

Activity II: Discuss the following "Ten Warning Signs"[3] of Alzheimer's disease. When are some situations "normal," and when are some not? Use it as a checklist to help you know who may exhibit some of the symptoms. Talk with a physician, find a support group, and try to communicate with the older person.

Ten Warning Sings of Alzheimer's Disease

◆Recent memory loss that affects functioning—forgetting more than the person remembers; repeating the same question and not remembering either the answer or having asked the question

◆Difficulty performing familiar tasks—preparing a meal and forgetting to serve it or forgetting they prepared it

◆Problems with language—forgetting simple words and substituting inappropriate ones that make the sentence incomprehensible

◆Disorientation of time and place—the person becomes lost on his/her own street or does not know where or how he/she got to a particular location

◆Poor or decreased judgment—forgetting to watch a child and leaving the house to do something else

◆Problems with abstract thinking—inability to balance a checkbook or figure out a solution

◆Misplacing things—putting things in inappropriate places, such as an iron in the refrigerator, and not being able to locate them

◆Changes in mood or behavior—experiencing rapid mood swings for no apparent reason

◆Changes in personality—drastic changes, often becoming extremely irritable, suspicious, or fearful

◆Loss of initiative—becoming very passive, requiring prompting to get involved in activities

Further Exploration

Exploration I: Make sure you have lists—names, addresses, and phone numbers—of your parents' physicians. Know where insurance cards are. Be aware of what medications they may be taking, and check for possible side effects or interactions. Stay informed of physical and mental changes occurring with your parents.

Exploration II: Become aware of local Alzheimer's disease associations in your community. The organizations can use your help as a volunteer or to support ongoing research and legislative issues.

Exploration III: Prevention is still the best cure. Take care of yourself—and encourage your parents to do so—with regular check-ups, a healthy diet, and moderate exercise.

Notes

[1]Monica Blumenthal, AARP's "Caring & Coping," 1991, 5. (booklet)
    [2]Nancy L. Mace and Peter V. Rabins, M.D. *The 36-Hour Day* (Baltimore: Johns Hopkins Press, 1981).
    [3]Information adapted from "Is it Alzheimer's? Ten Warning Signs," the National Alzheimer's Association.

Chapter 4

Intervening for Parents

Mother's fall occurred almost a year after her heart attack. After the fall, her situation began to change quickly in the months that followed. There were numerous visits for various medical services: physical therapy, cataract surgery, hearing aids, urinary tract treatments. During the same time period, her arthritis worsened, as did her confusion.

For several months she had a sitter from a private duty service during the day, and we hired a woman to prepare her dinner meals and stay with her through breakfast. Meals-On-Wheels delivered lunch each weekday. Our family provided transportation to doctors' offices and the hairdresser. Necessarily, I began helping her with check writing and the taxes.

The need for me to intervene became increasingly apparent. Mother let the day help go, insisting she could not afford it. Because she was no longer permitted to walk alone when she went outside the house, she became lonely and depressed. Mother complained about the night woman, and I often found moldy leftovers in the refrigerator. The smoke alarm went off when Mother forgot she had left beans cooking on the stove. Paint peeled, gutters leaked, and the yard was overgrown. She fretted over paperwork and became agitated that she did not have enough money to live on, that the house no longer belonged to her, and that I was going to put her out on the street. In some instances, she was not able to recognize her brother-in-law and old friends.

At times during the day it was hard to rouse her, and often she was confused and forgetful. Yet, Mother refused to do anything to change her situation, and I, her child, felt powerless. Many times I left her house in fear, fury, frustration, or quiet desperation, knowing that something had to change and not knowing how to initiate it. The decision, however, was not one I was *able* to make. After spending my entire life listening to, rebelling against, or consciously ignoring her relentless directives, I could not reverse the roles quite so quickly. She was still my mother.

On one of the many mornings that she would call me to come over before work, the conversation began with the usual rhythm: "I could not sleep at all last night for worrying . . ." Her worries were that she had no money and no place to go. Stricken by the wild look in her tense face, I backed toward the car. "I have to go to work now. I will call you." As soon as I arrived at work, I called her financial advisor.

"Do you have power of attorney?" he asked.

"No."

"Get it," was his terse reply.

My mother finished college at the beginning of the Depression. She watched her family lose home and livelihood. She pulled us through some difficult financial decisions my father had made. Mother had been a shrewd businesswoman on a teacher's salary for more years than I had been alive. I, on the other hand, was never too far from being broke. While earlier in life she would have never trusted me with her finances, I was now more capable of handling them than she was in her condition. *Right.*

In order to take on such a responsibility, I had to get my life in some sort of order. No more excuses. Be more responsible. I began by giving up the struggling advertising business, and took a full-time position—which involved some traveling—and then moved to another neighborhood. Not long after our move, Mother decided to move into a retirement center.

Role Reversal

Stepping into a parenting role for your mother or father is a difficult thing to do. We have been taught to respect our parents and to look to them as our authority figures and role models. Reversing the roles can be quite threatening.

The question about power of attorney, however, caught my attention. The meaning of the word "power" is the ability to act or do and refers to empowerment. Power of attorney gives one person the right to act on behalf of another.

Part of the role reversal process was giving myself permission to have authority; power to make decisions and to bear the consequences. I could no longer hide behind any one person, maintain my sense of innocence, or assume a hands-off attitude. My responsibility was to *act* and to *do* on behalf of my mother.

Legal Reminders

The legal proceedings involved only a call to the attorney to activate the durable power of attorney Mother had signed at an earlier date. Many of her assets had already been placed jointly in our names. Being prepared made this juncture easier for us both.

The issue of incompetence occurs in the absence of such preparations. When a person is incompetent to care for his or her affairs, various legal proceedings can be instituted. *Conservatorship*, or "guardianship of property", gives another person or institution the right to manage the individual's financial affairs. This is a court process that can incur costly legal fees and take several months. "Guardianship of person" is similar to conservatorship but concerns managing the physical care of the person who might be refusing needed care. This is also a court process, again often lengthy and involved. Since these processes differ from state to state, they should be thoroughly investigated with an attorney.

The best strategy in caring for aging parents is to plan together. Talk through options with them and their attorney and financial advisor earlier in the process rather than later. Try to insure that three basic documents are in place: an up-to-date will, a durable power of attorney, and a living will—advanced medical directives policy—or health care power of attorney. Know where these documents are located. On file in the attorney's office is often the safest, most convenient place for a will and other important documents.

Another legal and financial matter to investigate is the way a caregiver can transfer assets. A parent can give a certain amount of money—usually $10,000—in a single year to a child without incurring any gift tax. For large estates—over $100,000—establishing a trust can have tax and probate advantages.

Some families also try the "spend down" theory. The goal is to get the older person's resources under $2,000 in order to qualify for Medicaid: state medical assistance programs. State laws vary, however, and the child's personal finances can be investigated for any assets that may have been transferred by the parent during the past three years. Again, consult an attorney—preferably one knowledgeable about issues of the aging—before you act.

Community Resources

Investigate what help is available for older persons in the community. In most areas there are senior action centers and Meals-on-Wheels programs. Social groups and telephone networks can help to keep older persons involved in life, even if their activities are limited.

The telephone book, churches, and hospitals are good places to start to identify resources. Local chapters of various national organizations, such as the Alzheimers' Association, provide literature and other resources, as well as support groups that can be beneficial to the caregiver. (See Appendix for listing of national resources.)

In some communities Volunteer Caregivers Networks have begun. These programs—partially funded by grants—can provide needed transportation, meals, and coordination of other services available in the area. Programs such as Friendly Visitors and Adopt-a-Grandparent send volunteers on a weekly basis to spend time with shut-ins.

Continuum of Care

Continuum of care is a term most people have become acquainted with through the nation's health care reform movement. Care should be provided to an individual at the most appropriate level and at the most effective cost. Applying this concept to aging parents can be helpful in gauging when and how to intervene.

Independent Living

Ask any older person what he or she wants for the rest of life and likely you will get the answer: "Stay in my own home and be as independent as possible, as long as possible." This was the answer given to a researcher when he surveyed over 35,000 retirees across America. He then designed the concept of *Independent Living Club of America*®. (See Appendix B)

A range of services—house and yard maintenance, cleaning, meal delivery, transportation, emergency response systems, and priority access to nursing home care—can be purchased at discounted rates and from reliable vendors through the "club," helping older persons maintain their independence. Senior networks similar to this and other pilot programs (often federally funded) are beginning in many communities in an effort to find workable solutions for the increasing number of aging Americans.

Care managers are also available in some areas. For a fee, care managers help family members work out a care plan and assist in finding resources to meet the older person's needs such as check writing or finding transportation. These professionals can also be instrumental in helping resolve family conflicts and assisting adult children who live geographically distant from their aging parents.

Out-of-home Care

Some communities have day care centers or programs for senior citizens. These centers provide socialization for the aging parent, respite care for the caregiver, and care while family members are at work.

Other options for short-term, out-of-home care are also available. Nursing homes, hospitals, boarding homes, and foster homes provide respite for caregivers or care for the older person while other family members go on vacation.

Home Care

A variety of services are available in the home, from companion care and home-delivered walkers to skilled nursing. Some of the options to consider are:

- *Companion, sitter, or homemaker*: This service is available on a continuous basis—usually in 8-hour shifts —for a variety of tasks: bathing, cooking, light housekeeping, and transportation. Services are usually paid for privately, at an average rate of ten to fifteen dollars per hour; the fee varies by geographic area.

- *Specialized equipment and adaptive devices*: Physical, occupational, and respiratory therapists from area hospitals can make home visits to evaluate the home setting and make recommendations to enhance the safety and comfort of the older person. Non-skid strips on floors and in tubs, hand rails and ramps, and devices such as button loops and flexible foot dressers can increase the independence of the older person. Specialized medical equipment —with an order signed by a doctor—is payable through Medicare Part B.

- *Skilled nursing, nursing assistants, therapists* (physical, occupational, speech, and respiratory), and *medical social services*: These services are provided by certified home care agencies; covered by Medicaid, Medicare (when appropriate criteria are met, especially homebound status and physician ordered for skilled, intermittent needs), and private insurance companies.

- *Hospice care:* Hospice is a special program, payable under the Medicare hospice benefit, for terminally ill patients—6-month prognosis determined by a physician—that supplies skilled nursing, nursing assistants, therapists, chaplains and bereavement services, medical social services, volunteers, medications, physician services, and in-patient respite care.

- *Respite care:* Primary caregivers are offered some relief in their continuous task through this service. Usually for two to four hour periods, a volunteer or professional comes into the home. Many organizations supply and underwrite the fee for respite care if it is not covered by insurance. Respite care can also be provided in out-of-home settings, as mentioned above.

Activities
◆Individually or in a group◆

Activity I: Study the following chart of Continuum of Long-term Care Services.[1] Think of an aging person you know and plot what type of care he or she needs with regard to housework, transportation, managing money, taking medication, eating dressing, bathing, and toileting. Discuss how this type of chart can help in making decisions about care services.

◆Continuum of Long-term Care Services◆

	Little or No Assistance	Moderate Assistance	Cannot Perform without Assistance
Home	x		
House sharing	x		
Home with chore service			
senior center	x	x	
nutrition service			
Retirement community	x	x	
Home with delivered meals			
homemaker/ aide		x	
boarding home telephone			

reassurance		
visiting		
Home with	x	x
adult day care		
Home with		
home care		
hospice care		x
respite care		
Continuing care		
community		x
(nursing care)		
Nursing home		x

Activity II: Often primary caregivers need help; many do not know they need help or do not know how to ask for it. Friends, neighbors, and relatives will often only see the older person on a "good" day and tend to minimize the stress placed on the caregiver. Take the following "Warning: Caregiver needs help!"[2] and be ready to help yourself or someone you love.

Warning: Caregiver Needs Help!

• Your relative's condition is worsening despite your best efforts. ____ YES ____NO ____Other

• No matter what you do, it is never enough.
____ YES ____NO ____Other

• You feel you are the only person in the world having to endure the situation. ____ YES ____NO ____Other

- You no longer have any time or place to be alone for even a brief respite. ____ YES ____NO ____Other

- Things you used to do occasionally to help out are now part of your daily routine. ____ YES ____NO ____Other

- Family relationships are breaking down because of the caregiving pressures. ____ YES ____NO ____Other

- Your caregiving duties are interfering with your work and social life to an unacceptable degree. ____ YES ____NO ____Other

- You are going on in a no-win situation just to avoid admitting failure. ____ YES ____NO ____Other

- You realize you are all alone and doing it all because you have shut out everyone who's offered help. ____ YES ____NO ____Other

- You refuse to think of yourself because "that would be selfish." ____ YES ____NO ____Other

- Your coping methods have become destructive: you are overeating/undereating, abusing drugs/alcohol, or taking it out on your relative. ____ YES ____NO ____Other

- There are no more happy times. Loving and caring have given way to exhaustion and resentment. You no longer feel good about yourself or take pride in what in what you are doing. ____ YES ____NO ____Other

Further Exploration

Exploration I: Imagine various scenarios of care options for your parent(s) when independent living is no longer possible. Try to really see yourself living with various alternatives in order to get a better understanding of what might be the best choice.

Exploration II: Having your own will current is good advice for adults of any age. Are your own affairs in order? Are provisions in place should your aging parent by chance outlive you?

Notes

[1]Based on "Spectrum of Long-term Care Services," one version widely adapted in the health care community.

[2]Adapted from John Wood, "Labors of Love," *Modern Maturity* (August-September, 1987) 31.

Chapter 5

Making Tough Decisions

My parents had been charter members when the retirement living center in our community was finally built. Their initial payment was made years before any construction began. Mother's best friend from college days was one of the first persons to move to the center. By taking this initiative, she was able to begin the remainder of her life in a new setting and became actively involved while still vibrant.

Mother never wanted to leave her house or the community she had lived in most of her life. Her church, bank, stores, sisters, and friends were all within a few blocks. The retirement center was "way out there," and she did not want to go live with "all those old people." For Mother, it was a kind of insurance for her, or last resort.

Whether it was from listening to my worries for her, listening to her friend who lived there, or maybe responding out of something from within, Mother finally agreed to move to the new personal care wing when it opened. There she would have her own room and bath, with meals in the hall dining room, medication supervision, personal assistance as needed, housekeeping, social activities, a beauty parlor, and physician services. If necessary, she would have primary access to the nursing care wing.

Mother, however, became immobilized. She could not plan or pack what she needed to take, much less clean out those things she would no longer be needing. Each time she tried to back out the last few weeks before her move, I was the one who could not let her. If this was not hard enough on me, I soon became the target for everyone's criticism: well-meaning family, neighbors, and friends. I was the focus of her own anger, fear, and frustration.

Saturday morning as we backed the U-Haul truck up to the front steps, Mother met us at the door, arms folded across her chest. "I'm sorry you've gone to all this trouble, because I'm *not* going," she said firmly.

We faltered mid-step, and then I took a deep breath and said, "Sure you are Mom; everything's ready." We then pushed past her and moved her belongings the rest of the morning.

She still did not go to the retirement center until the following Monday, 1 October, the day she had originally committed to. I met two cousins on my lunch hour, and we drove her out. Mother hesitated slightly with each step as she entered the teal carpeted corridor; she put on a bright smile and spoke to everyone she met down that long hall. We finally arrived at her apartment, the last one on the right.

"I made up my mind," she said, "that if I was coming out here, I would make myself talk and be friendly." I was proud of her, but also glad to leave her with my cousins to get her settled in.

After work I went back to her house to check for last-minute items. As I entered the silent house, it felt as though I was walking back in from the hospital after my father had died years ago. Perhaps it felt as if she had died or maybe she was just buried alive, and I had done it. Then

I cried. But there was the PTA open house to attend, and the children's soccer practice, piano lessons, dance, and the house to clean out and sell.

After days of going through her things, my dad's things that she had kept, my things for my entire pre-married life, I remarked that it would have been easier if she had died. People would have sent food, given me time off from work, been understanding and sympathetic.

Some of her belongings were given to family members, and I stored whatever I could ever use. After having two all-day Saturday yard sales, I sold the remaining junk to a flea-market dealer for $125, wondering all the while if I had done the right thing. When I went to make a last check on the house, its emptiness appalled me.

The fireplace and irons—both the brass ones in the living room and the wrought iron set in the den—were gone. The vacant spots where the stove and refrigerator had been nearly all my life changed the shape of the room. I glanced one last time and noticed the worn, patterned linoleum, the bare pine shelves in the paneled den, and the echoing bathrooms and hollow closets.

And then, I remembered: *"Oh, no! I forgot to empty the garment bag that had my Brownie and Girl Scout uniforms, my first dance recital costume, my junior bridesmaid's dress from my cousin's wedding. Gone! With the mismatched dishes and odd linen."* Again, I cried.

When I arrived home, Mother called. She knew I had been crying and asked why. Since I could not tell her that her house was gone—I had sheltered her from that information—I only said, "Just everything." She understood and said, "You're tired. Go to bed. It will be all right." Her words were my consolation. At that moment she was again what she had always been to me: my mother. She was happy, relatively; and life continues.

When a Move Is Necessary

Sometimes it becomes impossible or impractical for aging parents to remain in their homes. Perhaps the expense and maintenance of a house has become unmanageable. Maybe there are no longer neighbors living near them, or opportunities for socialization have diminished. Safety is an important issue in deciding whether aging parents should remain in their home.

Moving to an apartment, where independence can be maintained on a smaller scale, is one option. A boarding home, personal care home, or congregate living situation are other possible options. Many apartment or condominium complexes become naturally occurring retirement communities because maintenance responsibilities are lessened. Older residents tend to look after one another—sharing rides and food, taking walks, and checking on each other daily by phone or visit—and take pride in the independence of the group. This may be an intermediate move if more nursing care is needed later.

The older person, however, must be willing to take active steps in making such a move: giving up the familiar home and possessions and making the commitment to relocate, even if it is in the same neighborhood. Researchers have found that the most common mistake older persons make is waiting too long. The longer they wait, the harder it is to relocate and the less chance there will be for successful move. Making a change requires energy. Too often older people think, "I'll wait 'til I really need it," and

then have too little left—physically, mentally, emotionally—
to invest in any new beginning.

Scenarios to Consider

Scenario One: Mother's college roommate, while in her
mid-seventies, commandeered the selling of her home and
the distribution of possessions she would not need. She
then chose the premier location and decor of an apartment
at the new retirement community and moved across town
where she could (1) be assured of continuing care, (2)
become actively involved in the life and leadership of the
community there, and (3) still be living independently ten
years later.

Scenario Two: An aunt of mine gave up her home and
friends of twenty-five years on the west coast and moved
to a small apartment near her extended family. She, too,
was in her mid-seventies. In five short years, she endeared
herself to her family and her new community. When she
died, many mourned. She probably could not have chosen
a better way to live out her remaining years.

Scenario Three: Another aunt of mine continues to live
alone in her home of nearly fifty years. Her physical condition severely limits her activities, and she depends
heavily on her neighbors. They provide transportation,
bring her meals, and visit frequently. Periodically, she visits
with her daughters—who live out of state—and never
complains about anything. On Sundays when I visit her, I
am challenged to keep up with her mentally; she discusses
current events and keeps me informed of all the family
news.

All of the scenarios are viable solutions. For years I have wondered, "Why was my mother's situation not as viable?" "Why was it so painful?" I have felt anger and frustration and often wondered whether I was somehow at fault. In retrospect, my mother—whether from personality or dementia—could never have made the decision that her college roommate or sister made. Neither was she capable of remaining in her own home or of actively choosing any other option.

Mother's situation and choices were largely colored by the dementia. When I was going through her things after her death, I found a yellowed clipping. The clipping was from a syndicated newspaper column discussing the signs, symptoms, and curelessness of Alzheimer's disease. She always joked about her failing memory. I now wonder how long she lived with the real fear of her disease.

A dementia condition such as Alzheimer's requires twenty-four-hour care of the patient. I wish I had known more—more of the disease's manifestations and what to expect. Knowing this information could have minimized the anger and guilt and helped me deal with the fears—hers and mine. The stigma of such a disease often hinders diagnosis and education about it.

Because Mother needed twenty-four-hour care, and because providing it in the home setting seemed improbable—financially, emotionally, logistically—the retirement community with guaranteed nursing care access was the best option for us. Mother actually enjoyed some of it: the socialization and the lack of responsibility. She came to our home every Sunday. Three of her good buddies shared the same dining table with her at each meal, and she was given manicures for the first time in her life.

Many of the other residents, however, were more confused than Mother, who thought most of the activities were silly. She hated not being able to take her own medicine—even something like Pepto Bismal—without a doctor's order. I was bothered by the fact that there were no locks on residents' doors, and that Mother could not take a walk outside unless someone was with her. Of course, this was for her own safety. Staff members did not always communicate adequately with her what they were doing and why. They were good to her, though, and when I cried at her passing, it was with the staff members. They had been her family and mine for a crucial time period.

I often wondered whether Mother might have remained healthier if she had entered the retirement community earlier, when she was more independent and could have been more interactive with the residents. Entering earlier, however, was not something she could do. Many older persons have similar fears or constraints about leaving their homes, and often changing familiar circumstances contribute to a confused mental state.

The Myths of Medicare and Medicaid

Affording care was never the main worry in my mother's situation. Because she was fortunate to have savings for her later years, and because her condition was not prolonged, I did not have to contribute to her financial support. For many adult children, supplementing their parents' care is a major issue.

One great myth is that Medicare, or Medicaid, pays for nursing home care: yes and no. Defining what those programs actually cover and how to qualify are important considerations for you and your aging parent.

Medicare, which is available to anyone qualifying for Social Security, pays for *skilled services* whether in a home setting, hospital unit, or nursing home. Skilled services are specifically defined by Medicare. The older person must require the services of a registered nurse or therapist. Examples of such skilled services are intravenous injections, oxygen therapy, and rehabilitation (physical, speech, or occupational therapy).

Personal, custodial, or intermediate care is not covered by Medicare. Other limitations apply such as requiring the patient to be hospitalized for at least three days before being discharged to a skilled nursing facility. Also, only a limited number of days (100) is payable, even though other conditions are met. There is also a co-payment after the first twenty-one days. The nursing home must be licensed and participate in the Medicare program. In actuality, Medicare rarely pays for nursing home care, except in limited and specific circumstances.

Medicaid, the state-funded medical assistance program, differs state by state. Basically, the older person cannot have resources greater than $2,000. When both partners are still living, however, allowance is made so that one can receive assistance without impoverishing the other.

Significant transfer of resources within thirty-six months of the older person's entry into the nursing facility can affect how Medicaid is granted. If eligibility is met, Medicaid covers both intermediate and skilled nursing care. Nursing facilities, however, can choose their degree of participation in the Medicaid program, and beds are often scarce. Someone on a list for a Medicaid bed can wait a year or more.

Most private insurance will not cover nursing home care; be careful when purchasing such a policy. Consult a financial expert with knowledge in the area, and consider the following:

- Does the policy cover any nursing home cost or only skilled nursing care? Does it require prior hospitalization?
- Can the insurer cancel the policy only for non-payment of premiums?
- Is there realistic inflation protection?
- What is the length of time pre-existing conditions are excluded?
- Are there permanent exclusions for certain conditions such as Alzheimer's disease?

Choosing a Nursing Home

Approximately 20,000 nursing homes in our country provide care for about 5 percent of the older population. Recent statistics predict that 40 to 45 percent of those turning age 65 (in 1993) will stay in a nursing home at least once. Half of these will stay less than six months, one in five will stay a year or more, and one in ten will stay more than three years.

The Long-Term Care Ombudsman Program is a federally required part of each state agency on aging. Ombudsmen regularly visit nursing homes in their areas and investigate complaints. They provide the public with helpful information.

Hospital discharge planners or social workers, your parent's physician, or care managers can help determine the type or level of care needed. They can explain what services certain facilities provide and make recommendations for present and future needs.

The three levels of care in long-term facilities are:

- *Personal care*—sometimes called assisted living—provides medication and other supervision; assistance with bathing, dressing, and grooming; meals; and supervised activities. Medicare and Medicaid do not cover personal care.

- *Intermediate care* provides twenty-four-hour nursing supervision and assistance with all needs, medical or social. Many patients may be seriously ill and die and yet only need intermediate, or continuous nursing care. Medicaid addresses intermediate care; Medicare does not.

- *Skilled care* provides the services of a registered nurse or therapist for such needs as intravenous injections, oxygen therapies, or dressing changes. Both Medicare and Medicaid cover skilled nursing care when specific regulations are met.

Use the following questions as a guide in choosing a nursing home.

- Does it have a good reputation in the community?
- Does it have a list of references?
- Is it convenient for family and friends to visit?
- Is it certified for Medicare and/or Medicaid?
- What are the admission requirements for residents?

Activities
◆Individually or in a group◆

Activity I: Discuss what other things you should consider in choosing a nursing home. Invite your area ombudsman to talk with your church or community group.

Activity II: Project a time when you will visit parents in a nursing home and plan what you would do. Brainstorm activities that could make the time meaningful for you and your parent. Also, come up with list of useful and interesting gifts for a nursing home resident.

Further Exploration

Exploration I: Visit (with your parent, if possible) nursing homes in your area. Talk with residents as well as staff. Make unscheduled visits; visit at meal times.

Exploration II: If your parent goes to a nursing home, get involved in residence councils. Educate the staff on who your parents are, what they were like in younger years, and what they need now.

Exploration III: As appropriate, help your parents begin to give away possessions (or at least put a name on an item). Rather than being morbid, it can be a meaningful opportunity and a tremendous service.

Chapter 6

Receiving
Needed Consolation

For the next fifteen months I drove to the care center every
Sunday to pick up Mother. She would introduce me to the
same bent people, ask me about the children and work,
and quiz me about her business affairs. I could hear her as
I was leaving proudly telling her friends, "That tall, lanky
gal is my daughter." *I love you, too, Mother. Why could we
never say it to each other?*

During December of the same year, I noticed another
change in Mother's behavior. One Sunday I found her dis-
traught over trying to write Christmas cards. "I can't do
it!" she cried.

She was not only unable to do the handwriting, but
also the thought processes that went with the writing and
addressing. I told her that it did not really matter, no one
expected cards from her, and that I never had the time to
send cards myself. This, however, was not comforting to
Mother. She kept saying, "I'm losing my mind. They're
going to take me to the mental hospital." Her terror was
obvious. We went to the doctor the next day, and for the
first time I heard her condition referred to as Alzheimer's.

On Christmas Eve, Mother did not know why I was there to pick her up or why she was going to my house. Christmas Day, when my cousin arrived to pick her up, she was not dressed and was unable to understand why Sara Ann was giving her a present. The next month everyone was amazed how rapidly her condition declined. She could no longer dress herself, struggled to walk, and refused to go to meals. Mother was unable to tell anyone where she was living and often would not leave the bed. She called many times a day, telling me her stockings were too tight for her legs, she had outgrown her underwear and clothes, and that she was out of the *Depend*® pads she used regularly. Still trying, I bought queen size hose for her small legs, a new set of underwear, several new loose dresses, and sixty-count packages of *Depend*® pads.

"Go in there and get stuff out of her drawers and wrap it up, will you! Quit throwing away money!" a friend scolded me. When we finally cleaned out her belongings, we packed fourteen boxes of underwear and clothes, and found *Depend*® pads stuck in every possible cranny of her apartment. We also found pink packets of sweetener, wadded tissues, and peppermints in every pocket of clothing.

The difficulty Mother was having with her clothing, I found out later, was not that they were actually tight on her. The problem was that it became increasingly difficult for her to pull them up or fasten the hooks because of her failing strength. She was also having problems remembering where she left the clothing. I alerted the staff on personal care; they did their best caring for Mother that month—longer than they were required. All of us were surprised at the speed with which she decided to stop living.

When I returned from a short trip and went straight from the airport to see her, she was dressed and sitting on her sofa. She greeted me gratefully, "Oh, I'm so glad you made it." She then told me she had fallen and hurt her back and that she was dying. The nursing staff knew nothing about this; the doctor checked her and could find nothing wrong except some degenerative arthritis. I helped her into bed, sat in the chair beside her, and held her hand until she slept peacefully. Glancing across the room, I saw our reflection in the mirror, and it reminded me of sitting in intensive care with my father until his death. In retrospect, I felt as though I was doing the same kind of waiting, but this time with my mother.

In February I received the dreaded call from the care center that they were moving her to the nursing care wing. All my life Mother had drilled me to never, never put her in a nursing home. Rationally I knew it was the only thing to do, but emotionally I felt like a criminal. I found it especially hard when she begged to go home with me everyday. I realized what she wanted was a safe place to die.

During the earlier stages of her illness, we looked for a larger house. I had taken her with me to see a four-bedroom house a few blocks from her home. The house had a large room across the back of the first floor with a bathroom and wet bar that could be converted to a kitchenette. When I suggested that we all move there and find help during the day when she was alone, she told me forcefully that she would never live with us. So we bought a brick townhouse without a downstairs bedroom.

Still, I continued to conceive of ways in which she could stay in our home. One solution, I thought, would be to use nurses around the clock. This time my husband intervened. "You can't do it," he said. "It almost killed you before, and this is worse. You can't do it."

Over the next several months, I would leave work, stop to eat with my children and husband, and then drive to the nursing home to see Mother. I remember many nights leaving at 10:30 or 11:00 P.M., and wondering how in my night blindness and fatigue I ever made it home safely. I also remember feeling a deep sense of guilt. I had to live so much on the surface when life was calling me to the depths.

Mother continued to die at a rapid pace. One Sunday, the children and I went directly from church to the nursing home. As we passed the nursing station, I noticed a nurse smiling at us and nodding at an old woman strapped in a wheel chair nearby. "She's glad to see you," she said.

I looked again at the old woman, who focused on me with a gaping smile and whose neck was crooked back nearly ninety degrees. I had not recognized my own mother.

"What's with the neck thing?" I whispered to the nurse, hoping the children would not be afraid.

"The doctor says it is just another manifestation of the Alzheimer's," she said.

We rolled her out to the sun porch, but she was agitated and frightened of the open spaces. During the later stages she often saw shadowy figures in the air, and "things" tried to harm her. Mother also talked to people we could not see and was terrified of the large chrome whirlpool they put her in once a week.

Mother then quit eating. Her sisters and her best friend visited her on numerous occasions during her last days. On 1 May at 6:00 A.M., after ten days in a near coma, Mother died. I was with her that night, and I do not remember her completely losing consciousness. Sometime between four and five in the morning, she fixed her gaze on me and did not waver. *What was that about?* I have asked myself that question a thousand times.

Mother finally closed her eyes; her breathing became mechanical, like the sound of a car engine dying. Four breaths pattern, *ha-ha-ha-ha-he;* then three, *ha-ha-ha-he;* then two . . . and then one. I found myself listening intently. I strained. Then nothing.

"You did real good," I whispered fiercely, stroking her hair and lightly kissing her forehead. Then I sobbed, not just because she was gone, but for the terrible finality that death leaves to those behind.

The Comfort of Strangers

My mother's family had always been very close. Rarely did I remember her making a decision without conferring with at least three of her sisters. Trusting anyone outside her family network was difficult for Mother.

Going to the retirement community was like going to a far country; she feared strangers would not meet her needs there. As her illness progressed, I found myself needing more and more emotional distance from the situation just to survive. In thinking back, I recall numerous blessings we each received from "strangers." Sometimes we are too involved to provide the best help. Maybe that is part of our forgiveness work. We can help others in ways that we could not help ourselves and our families.

The hospice movement in our country has established a wonderful network of "strangers" who provide care to the dying and their families. These nurses, social workers, therapists, chaplains, and volunteers minister in specially trained ways. They can address and help ease much of the fear surrounding the dying process by anticipating needs and encouraging communication. Though we did not have hospice care, I was blessed through the book *Final Gifts.*[1]

In *Final Gifts,* two hospice nurses share their knowledge of ways in which the dying communicate. In reading their work, I realized my mother left me some words about her departure. We remembered her talking peacefully about the gray horse running around outside and sticking his head in through the window by her bed. My daughter told me about Marmee staring at the ceiling and seeing her brothers and sisters playing in the fields. I recalled her looking out the window and laughing, "That little calf just jumped over the fence." From these words I take comfort in knowing that she was seeing familiar surroundings as she moved on. I hope she is playing in safe pastures she knew as a child.

Processing Your Grief

Local hospice groups—identifiable through the National Hospice Organization—provide chaplains, bereavement coordinators, and social workers who can help you work through the grief process. These trained professionals can talk with you individually or in a group. The hospice program offers bereavement support to family members for a year after the death of a hospice patient. (These groups are often open to the community at large as well.)

Hospital chaplains and social workers are good resources for help in the grieving process. They, too, can provide support, and can refer you to other available sources in your community. Ministers, counselors, funeral directors, and spiritual directors are additional options.

Activities
◆Individually or in a group◆

Activity I: Share in your small group any experiences you have had with a parent dying. What were some of your feelings? How has guilt and forgiveness been experienced in your situation?

Activity II: Share in your small group ways in which you process your grief. Consider the following activities:

(1) Visit the grave site and talk to your loved one.
(2) Talk to family members and friends who knew the loved one well.
(3) Write about the loved one and your feelings for him or her.

Activity II: As appropriate, determine your parents' wishes for their funerals. Often they will be more comfortable knowing that they have communicated what they want to you. If your parents are unable or unwilling to do this with you now, remember that funerals are for the living and do what is best for you. Talking with a funeral director ahead of time can help make a difficult time easier.

Further Exploration

Exploration I: Read *Final Gifts*. (Bibliographic information provided in Appendix.)

Notes

[1]Maggie Callanan, *Final Gifts* (New York: Bantam Books, 1992).

Chapter 7

Owning Your Forgiveness

I was going to the beach—my place of escape—with my husband and children. Though worried about leaving my mother, I went anyway. I remember playing in the water, relaxing in the warmth of the sun, enjoying myself, and feeling free. The time was brief, and we then we went back home. I went to my room to unpack. When I opened a dresser drawer, I found Mother lying in her pink rayon pajamas, dead, as though she was in her coffin. It was my punishment for having any time for myself.

The months that followed Mother's death were filled with these haunting dreams. In one of the dreams, Mother had come out of her coma and was wanting to go back to her house, which had already been sold. Painful feelings take a long time to heal.

Immediately following her death, I felt a sense of relief. There was closure to so many of the unknowns. The slow and painful process had not lasted indefinitely. She was in a better place. We could all move on with our lives. Right? I found that it was not as easy as it seemed.

The changes happened so quickly. Mother had gone from being the strongest force in my life to someone I barely knew. All of these changes happened in the span of three-and-a-half years. At age 38, I felt like a failure.

My coping skills have always been one of my strongest features. I manage well under multiple challenges, usually with a smile. I got through those years because I *had* to, because people depended on me, and because long ago I had learned to separate pain and store it somewhere deep inside.

Instead of moving on with my life after Mother's death, I felt inertia. I *kept* on, because life continues to move on; responsibilities remain. The need to spend time looking deeper within became apparent.

My sense of failure was centered on the fact that I was unable to keep this terrible thing from happening to Mother. I could do nothing to stop the process, and I felt she expected me to do this. She did not "go gentle into that good night." Whether it was her disease or her own tenacious personality, she did not welcome old age and death. When things did not work as they had before—whether it was her eyesight, hearing, or her sense of control—Mother became very frustrated. She was never one to sit back and contemplate the life she had lived and ponder about the life beyond; she may have been too afraid to do so. Unlike my aunt, who picked out her coffin and wrote her own obituary, Mother was unable to talk about her death. She never verbalized to me any comforting visions of eternity.

The only thing I could do for her was to be with her during her last hours. I did not know what to say or how to help her. Her friend had said, "I think she's waiting for you to tell her something." *What? What could I say in the last hours of her life, when we had not been able to really communicate in years?* I remember saying something generic: "I love you. Don't worry. We'll be fine." Then I talked for some time about the children, feeling hopelessly inadequate to address her fears or my own.

During the long drive home from the nursing home each night, I listened to a Carly Simon song, "Life Is Eternal." It is based on the words of Rossiter Worthington Raymond (1840–1918):

> *Life is eternal,*
> *and love is immortal,*
> *and death is only a horizon,*
> *and a horizon is nothing*
> *save the limit of our sight.*

For a long time, I was unable to see past the horizon. Life seemed too hard, the prognosis too grim. *I mean, if we are all just going to die anyway?* With her death, I saw the end of my life too. How could I go on finding meaning and joy each day in the face of death?

When I look in the mirror, I see my mother. Whether or not she could express faith about dying, she certainly taught me about living. She showed me that we age on the outside, but we never really notice the differences inside. She also taught me that time moves on so superficially, and that the only viable response to life is to live it the best way that we can. That is all any of us can do.

Setting healthy boundaries was helpful whenever I found myself asking the questions, "How could I have done it differently?" "How could it have been better?" I finally gave myself permission to stop re-evaluating or re-playing the scenario. Each individual deals with grief in his or her own way; every situation is in need of its own unique grace. What we can never quite forget, maybe we

can come closer to forgiving—even ourselves. By the grace
of God, that is enough.

Activities

Activity I: Write your final conversation with your
parent(s) in the way you would choose. If you did not
receive the blessing you would have liked from your parents, write your own now.

Activity II: As you can, help someone else. Whether you
take an elderly neighbor to the grocery store or volunteer
at a local nursing home or hospital, you can help someone
else who is struggling by simply sharing your story.

Afterword

Many stories have been told about my birth. A cousin wrote me after Mother's death and told me that she would always remember my mother sitting on a stool at grandmother's feet, telling Granny she was pregnant with me: Mother laughed and laughed. Other family members also laughed when they heard the news, calling my parents "Abraham and Sarah." Relatives from both sides of my large extended family gathered at the hospital the day I was born.

Isaac was born to Abraham and Sarah; the name Isaac means "laughter." My names mean "gift from God" and "truthful one."

So these days, especially when I write, I am telling the truth. My gift is trying to put into words what others are feeling.

Maybe it is not too late to laugh either.

Appendix A: Answers

Chapter 1

Answers to Palmore's Fact vs. Myth Aging Quiz:

1.	F	12.	T
2.	T	13.	F
3.	F	14.	T
4.	T	15.	F
5.	F	16.	T
6.	T	17.	F
7.	F	18.	T
8.	T	19.	F
9.	F	20.	T
10.	T	21.	F
11.	F	22.	T

Appendix B: National Organizations

◆**Alzheimer's Association**
919 N. Michigan Avenue, Suite 1000
Chicago, IL 60611
(312) 853-3060

Provides free informational literature and location of closest local chapter.

◆**American Association of Retired Persons**
601 E Street NW
Washington, DC 20049
(202) 434-2277

Many helpful publications are available at no cost, including information on financial planning and long-term care insurance.

◆*Independent Livng Club of America*®
300 Pettigru Street
Greenville, South Carolina 29601

The *Independent Living Club of America*® was developed by Wilson Worley, National Retirement Corporation, Greenville, South Carolina. The concept was market-tested in the Baltimore, Maryland, area.

◆**National Association of Area Agencies on Aging**
1112 16th Street NW, Suite 100
Washington, DC 20036
(202) 296-8130

Provides information on location and phone number of the agency in your area for social and medical services.

♦National Association of Private Geriatric Care Managers
655 N. Alvernon Way, Suite 108
Tucson, AZ 85711
(602) 881-8008

Offers a list of private geriatric care managers.

♦National Hospice Organization
1901 N. Moore Street, Suite 901
Arlington, VA 22209
(800) 658-8898

Supplies information about hospice benefits and local hospice organizations.

Appendix C: Suggested Reading

Callanan, Maggie, and Kelley, Patricia. *Final Gifts*. New York: Bantam Books, 1992.

Carter, Rosalynn. *Helping Yourself Help Others*. New York: Random House, 1994.

Cox, Barbara J., and Waller, Lois Lord. *Bridging the Communication Gap with the Elderly: Practical Strategies for Caregivers*. Chicago: American Hospital Publishing, 1991.

Greenberg, Vivian. *Your Best Is Good Enough: Aging Parents and Your Emotions*. Lexington MA: Lexington Books, 1989.

Jackson, Billie. *The Caregivers Roller Coaster: A Practical Guide to Caring for the Frail Elderly*. Chicago: Loyola University Press, 1993.

Lester, Andrew D., and Lester, Judith L. *Understanding Aging Parents*. Philadelphia: Westminster Press, 1980.

Mace, Nancy L. and Peter V. Rabins, M.D. *The 36-Hour Day*. Baltimore: Johns Hopkins Press, 1981.

Munsch, Robert. *Love You Forever*. Ontario: Firefly Books Ltd., 1986.

Pritikin, Enid, and Reece, Trudy. *Parentcare Survival Guide*. New York: Barrons, 1993.